FITSTYLE YOUR LIFE

ABOUT ZOEFIT

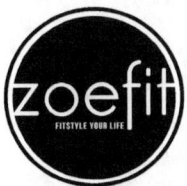

The origin of "zoe" (pronounced ZOH-ee) comes from Greek meaning life or the state of one who is possessed of vitality. Fit is short for the word fitness. Life and fitness are inextricably linked. Just like in the company name.

www.zoefit.com

www.ingramcontent.com/pod-product-compliance
Lightning Source LLC
Chambersburg PA
CBHW060346290526
45791CB00004B/1548

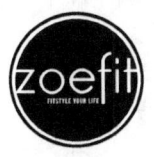

FitStyle
YOUR LIFE

5 Simple Keys
for Taking Exercise
off Your To-Do List

SHANA N. SCHNEIDER

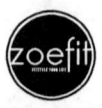

www.zoefit.com

SPECIAL THANKS

A HUGE thank you goes to my husband.
My Mom and Dad. My Sister. My Great Aunt.
Christie Cole. Michelle Claudnic. Naomi Taylor.
Sharon Kunz. Tracy Edwards. Janice Kaplan.
Roxanne Coady. Lisa Kimmel. Kimberly Muller.
Anees Chagpar. Karen Giaquinto. Susan Abramson.
Rob Bettigole (especially for the 10x10x10 Challenge).
Sarah Aldrich. Claire Criscuolo. Sonia Baghdady.
Shelly Saczynski. Alena Gribskov. Jim Boyle. Rick Hunt.
Astrid Gufler. Don Filer. Shana Gauvrit. Shana Ross.
All the FITWEEK/ZoeFit subscribers!

**And You. I know you didn't have to
open this book, but you did.**

CONTENTS

INTRODUCTION

Fitness is fundamental to keeping us healthy. We know the statistics about the physical and emotional benefits of exercise, but we still don't do it or stick to our goals — until now.

I'm going to challenge you to let go of some of the preconceptions you have about exercise and what it means to get fit. The key to getting and staying fit is learning how to bring fitness into your everyday life. I know; it seems obvious, right? And you may be asking yourself, exactly how do I go about doing this? Well, that's where my method of "FitStyling" comes in.

This is a practical guide to FitStyle Your Life. I think of it as a "mini mani," or a miniature manifesto. It outlines the five keys I've used to take exercise off my to-do list and make it part of my everyday life. Fitness is my lifestyle. Yep, I've dropped the guilt from my schedule; I'm done feeling like I just don't have enough hours in the day. And that's not because my schedule is predictable or because I've found some secret to adding a 25th hour to my day.

By the time you finish, I hope you'll share some of the insights I've gathered so fitness becomes attainable for you, in a way that won't take any additional time out of your day. And you'll have the tools to be the guilt-free, fittest you that you can be.

The "FitStyle Your Life" approach has 5 keys:

1. Stand up for your own good.
2. Make every second count.
3. Enjoy yourself.
4. Stage your living spaces.
5. Be thankful.

I'll take you through each one so that you can start to put these in place for yourself.

This is about creating a lifestyle. It's not an add-on or something for you to try to fit into your schedule. It's part of how you think, move, and live. I try to look at it this way. Think about Lady Gaga or Bette Midler. Their style is so over the top. When they perform or make an appearance, you expect to see something outrageous. That's not because they've done it once or twice; it's because they do it regularly.

Maybe there's a friend of yours or a co-worker who shows up in outfits that make you say to yourself, "I like her style." That's because "style" is doing something habitually. Doing something once or a few times doesn't make it your style. That's why, when it comes to fitness, we need to make it something we do everyday — something people come to expect from us and something we come to expect of ourselves. And it's not as hard as you think! I promise.

TAKE THE CHALLENGE

Before you go any further, I want to give you a simple challenge. This is a great example of how you can bring fitness into your everyday life, too. It's the ZoeFit Abs Challenge. While you're reading this, I want you to engage your abdominal muscles.

If you're sitting right now, I want you to sit actively. Put both feet flat on the ground with your knees about hip-distance apart. You can do this same exercise standing up, too! Later on, you'll find out why that's important.

Now, suck in those abs, but not to the point where you can't breathe. We don't want you passing out! You want your abs pulled in and engaged. It should feel like when you cough or sneeze. In fact, do that. Give a little cough and see what it feels like. Can you see how your abs pull in like that?

Now, place one hand on the outside of your ribs and breathe in. Those ribs should go out laterally, pushing your hand slightly to the side. Then, when you breathe out, your hand goes back in. Now do that again, but put your hand on your stomach. When you breathe in and out your hand should barely move, because you're keeping your abs pulled in nice and tight.

By taking this abs challenge, you'll be doing a whole series of sit-ups and working on a flat stomach without having to get down on the floor or having anyone else even notice.

I'll throw in little reminders as we go along, too!

STAND UP FOR YOUR OWN GOOD

SITTING IS KILLING YOU.

Picture this. I'm sitting in my office at my computer, typing away. I'm fully into what I'm working on and have totally lost track of time. The next thing I know, the lights turn out and I'm sitting in the dark. At first I think, did the power go out? And then, I realize that no, my computer is still on. In fact, I had been sitting so still for so long that the motion detector determined no one was in the room. Has this ever happened to you?

What I want you to think about when you're sitting down is the fact you're giving that same message to your body. You're telling it, "Hey, no-one's moving around. Go ahead and shut down." When you're sitting for hours without getting up, you're telling your muscles that you don't need them. They can go ahead and shut down — and they will. What you don't see is that this inactivity causes an internal chain reaction. When our muscles aren't in use, they can't initiate the signals our bodies are looking for — telling it to breakdown fats and sugars. Instead, the build up throws our bodies out of whack. This is when you see an increase in risk for developing type 2 diabetes, cardiovascular disease, as well as a number of other health concerns. Oh, and those of you who make it to the gym or a fitness class, but still sit for hours on end each day — you're not in the clear. Studies are now showing that too much sitting will override the benefits of that one-hour workout. Physical inactivity can have devastating effects on the body. Period.

I found this visual helpful for me, so wanted to share it with you, too.

THIS IS YOUR BODY.

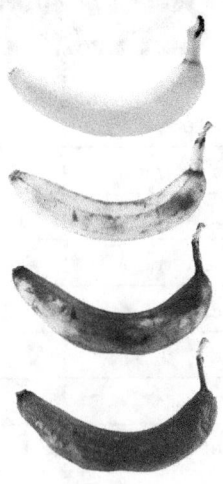

THIS IS YOUR BODY WITH EXCESSIVE SITTING OVER TIME (~4 OR MORE HOURS PER DAY).

How can we avoid this? This is where the first FitStyle key comes in. We simply need to stand up more!

Now, let me put in some context. Sitting for short periods like during a meal is fine. It's the hours on end that are the problem.

YOUR FITSTYLE PLAN

Take a few minutes to fill out the chart below. This will help you discover how much sitting you do throughout your day. Think about it — we don't just sit at the office. Maybe you have a long commute, or you collapse on the couch when you get home.

ACTIVITY	HOURS
Breakfast	
Commute	
Work/classes morning	
Lunch	
Work/classes afternoon	
Commute	
Dinner	
TV	
Computer at home	
Other	
TOTAL	

Compare your totals to the following:

- **Low risk** is sitting less than 3 hours a day in a chair or on a couch

- **Medium risk** is sitting 4-8 hours a day in a chair or on a couch

- **High risk** is sitting 8-11 hours a day in a chair or on a couch

We want to make sure we stay out of the high or medium risk zones. How are we going to get ourselves standing more?

Now, obviously you have to consider what your job allows you to do, but there are definitely ways to try to reduce the number of hours you spend sitting.

Here are a few ideas:

- **When people come to talk with you, stand up.** I've found it helps to keep distracting visits shorter and also eliminates that awkward feeling of: "I'm looking up at you while you're standing looking down talking to me." Try it, and I bet you'll feel like it makes more sense, too.

- **Use your phone as a reminder to stand up.** Whenever you pick up your phone or start looking at it, get up. (And if you're in the car, then you know you shouldn't be looking at your phone anyway, right?)

- **When somebody emails you at work, instead of emailing back, get up and go talk to them.** Plus, you'll get in some steps!

- **Ask yourself if you really need to take a seat.** So often, we sit down for no reason. We're constantly offered a seat when we're at the salon, dentist or a meeting. Next time, politely decline and take a stand instead!

We should have three curves in our back — the cervical curve (at the neck), the thoracic curve (at the shoulders), and the lumbar curve (at the lower back). You may be familiar with the lumbar curve if you've experienced lower back pain.

VERTEBRAL COLUMN

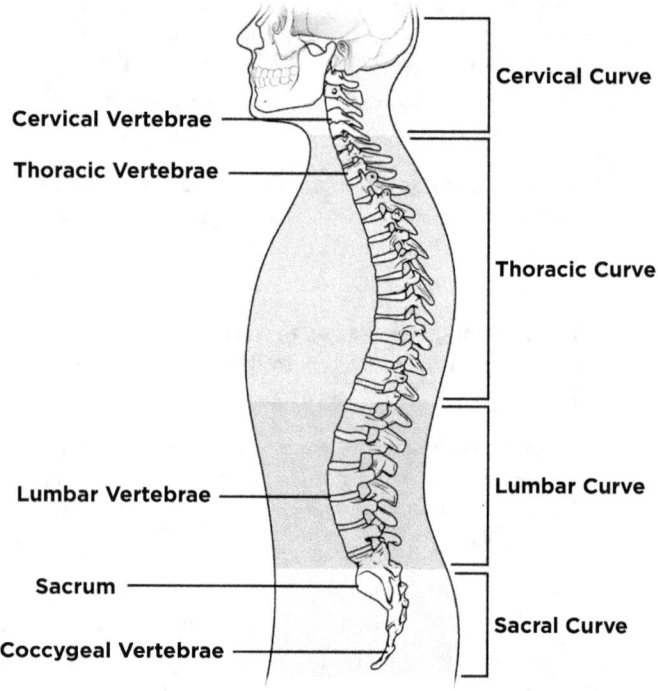

Cervical Curve

Cervical Vertebrae

Thoracic Vertebrae

Thoracic Curve

Lumbar Curve

Lumbar Vertebrae

Sacrum

Coccygeal Vertebrae

Sacral Curve

Those curves can get out of alignment, for example, when our head is too far forward or our hips are too far back. This will strain the back muscles and cause pain and discomfort over time. Many people suffer from lower back pain because of this. Sitting in chairs for too many hours can be a major culprit when it comes to throwing our posture out of whack.

So, here's what we're going to do.

YOUR FITSTYLE PLAN

If we're going to stand more, we need to know how to stand with good posture.

Follow these steps to find your sweet stance:

1. Stand with your feet parallel and about hip distance apart. Your weight should be evenly distributed across your toes and heels.

2. Slightly bend your knees, so they are relaxed and not locked.

3. Pull in your abs.

4. Relax your shoulders and pull them back just slightly. Let your arms hang at your sides.

5. Look straight ahead. Make sure your chin isn't forward or up.

Now, imagine a string coming out of the top of your head and pulling you up so you feel yourself getting lighter and maybe even a little taller. (This is honestly the only way I know to get that quick fix to look thinner and taller in no time flat!) We want to keep those lovely curves in our back, so try not to stand ramrod straight. Everyone is naturally curvy when we're talking about our spines.

Next, write down three ways you're going to stand up more during the day:

1. _____

2. _____

3. _____

Get a Post-it note, write these down, and put them in plain view until they become your style!

Lowering the number of hours that you're sitting throughout the day will have a significant impact on your fitness and, therefore, your health. This is the kind of low-hanging fruit that doesn't take any extra time or money to bring into your everyday life.

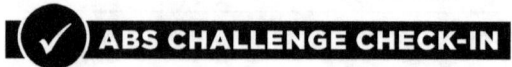

✓ ABS CHALLENGE CHECK-IN

How's that going? Are they still engaged?

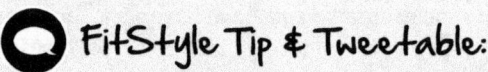

💬 FitStyle Tip & Tweetable:

Cats and dogs are, but chairs are not a 4-legged friend. Stand up for your own good! **#FITSTYLE**

BONUS TIP:
Three alternatives to sitting in a chair: the floor, a balance ball, and your own two feet! **#FITSTYLE**

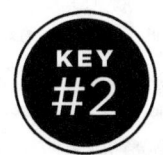

KEY
#2

MAKE EVERY SECOND COUNT

STOP LOOKING FOR A 25TH HOUR.

Let's just call out the elephant in the room right now. What do most people say is one of, if not the biggest, hurdles keeping them from exercising? It's that there just isn't enough time in the day. I know what you mean. When you think about how many hours you spend in the office or at work, plus any kind of commuting, plus preparing meals or other ways you spend your time before or after work, by the time you feel like you have a minute to stop, it's the end of the day and exercising may be the last thing you want to do — even though you know it would be good for you.

So, what if we changed how we look at making time for exercise? Typically, we think we need 30-minutes to an hour of dedicated time to exercise. Science is telling us otherwise. While general standards recommend we get 150-minutes of exercise per week or 30-minutes per day, it turns out those minutes don't need to be consecutive. What?! I know. Stay with me.

Here's the good news. 10-minute increments of moderate exercise done several times throughout our day can provide us with the same fitness benefits as slugging away at a workout for a whole hour straight, which most of us don't have in our regular schedules. But we do often have these short breaks throughout our day. It's also much easier to motivate ourselves to do something for just 10-minutes, knowing that at the end of it, we'll feel accomplished and successful!

Moderate activity during these breaks in our day is something any of us can achieve. What do I mean by moderate? It means you're increasing your heart rate, but probably not breaking a sweat. If you're walking, you're aiming for 100 steps per minute.

Now, the other aspect to consider is that while we may not have free time, we do have time. This is the key to making fitness an integral part of your life. We need to bring it into the activities that we're already doing during the day. Remember, any exercise you do is better than the exercise you're not doing at all!

There is a Chinese philosopher who said, "A thousand mile journey starts with the first step." And it's the same with fitness. This is not something you get to do in one take. Remember what we talked about at the beginning. We're creating a style for ourselves — a fitness lifestyle. It's something we do every day, and this style and perspective should permeate everything in our lives, including the choices we make.

The key is to focus on accumulated activity — not the hour or 30 minutes at one time, which you may or may not have each day. Why? Because it turns out that if you spend that time working out but are sedentary for the rest of the day, you lose all the benefit from having done that exercise! Crazy, but true.

By using this FitStyle key of making every second count, you'll start to realize there is an opportunity for fitness around every corner. For example, when I do laundry, instead of taking everything out of the dryer all at once (I do have a front loader; that's important to know!), I squat to pull 1-2 items out and put them on top, then I do it again until everything is out. In the short time it takes to unload the dryer, I've done at least one full set of squats!

Here are a few other examples:

- When I'm waiting for my popcorn to pop in the microwave, I'll do calf raises until the timer goes off.

- You can make standing in line an opportunity to work on balance by standing on one foot or targeting your legs by doing side leg lifts. (You can shift your weight subtly so no one will notice!)

- You can do plies while you're brushing your teeth.

These seem like small things, but they help you to create a fitness habit and style that will make a big impact on your health.

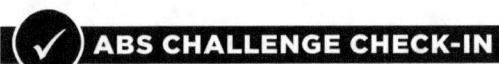 **ABS CHALLENGE CHECK-IN**

And this reminder matches perfectly with the topic. Keeping your abs engaged all day strengthens the stomach muscles without causing you to miss a beat or stop any of the other activities on your schedule!

YOUR FITSTYLE PLAN

Write down ways you can bring fitness into an everyday activity.

1. _____

2. _____

3. _____

Write down times during your day when you have 10-minutes and note how you can make those 10-minutes active.

1. _____

2. _____

3. _____

Think outside the box (or gym, in this case). If you take kids to rehearsals or sports practice, is there time when you're on the sidelines when you can get in some exercise?

What's great about FitStyling your life is that you can do it at any age, any fitness level, any time, and anywhere! It's part of your fitness continuum. If you love group fitness classes, like I do — I'm not gonna lie, sign me up for Zumba or Pilates any day! — this approach and mindset helps you fill in the gaps between classes. If your schedule is jam-packed and there is just no way anything else is getting into the mix, that's okay too, because you can bring fitness into what you're already doing.

So say goodbye to those days when you miss your workout and think, "Well, that's it. I guess this day is a fitness bust." When you make every second count, you have thousands of seconds each day to succeed!

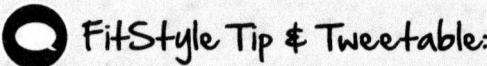 **FitStyle Tip & Tweetable:**

When you make every second count, you have thousands of seconds each day to succeed! **#FITSTYLE**

ENJOY YOURSELF

NO PAIN, NO GAIN? FORGET THAT.

Here's the thing. I do not get excited about something that's going to hurt, nor do I get motivated by the idea of enduring pain. It just doesn't do it for me. If anything, I'm more inclined to head in the opposite direction. If exercise is something we have a hard time doing, why would we be more inclined to do it with that kind of motto? I'd rewrite it this way. *If it's fun, then I'll run.*

Yep, it's true; getting exercise can be fun. I know some of you are probably shaking your head in disbelief, but here's the thing:

I'm a people person and I love to spend time with friends and family. This becomes another thing to work into my schedule on top of work and chores. Not that that's a bad thing, but I often saw it as a tradeoff with the time I have to exercise.

Here's what I want you to consider. Exercise doesn't have to be "alone time," separate from the people we want to spend time with or things we like to do. It can, in fact, be a lot of fun when you're hanging out with friends or with family. You can choose activities that get you all moving.

When I meet up with girlfriends for a ladies' night, we'll FitStyle it by finding some kind of fitness class none of us would want to go to by ourselves, like a belly dancing class or aerial silks, and then we have dinner afterwards.

While fitness can be done in a gym or studio, it doesn't have to be. I love to dance; I'll try any kind of dancing at least once. I have some friends who took me country line dancing. No one can tell me that isn't a workout. The number of steps you can rack up just trying to follow along to a few songs is phenomenal.

And have you seen the themed runs that are taking place all over the country? Remember how I said before — if it's fun, then I'll run? Well, these are great examples of events that fit the bill — there's the color run (where you get covered in color and look like a rainbow by the end of the course), the electric run (where you run through a course at night that's lit up with all kinds of cool displays), and the ugly sweater run (where you wear the ugliest sweater you can find, and people take this very seriously). These kinds of 5K runs, which aren't competitive, make for a fun experience you can talk about for ages. You can also choose to walk the course, so people at all different fitness levels can participate.

Keep things really simple. If you're catching up with a friend, instead of taking a seat at the coffee shop to sit and chat, look for high tables where you can stand up; or better yet, walk and talk.

The key is to mix fitness with things you enjoy, whether those are hobbies or the people you want to spend time with.

Maybe what you enjoy is binge-watching the latest series on Netflix. (I'll admit it. When *House of Cards* first came out, I watched the whole season in about two days. I did the same thing with season one of *Scandal*.) It's a guilty pleasure, but here's the thing: I've learned to activate that time by creating simple rules for watching. For example, when my favorite character comes on the screen, I'll do squats. Then when the scene changes, I'll do arm exercises. My family has a tradition of watching *White Christmas* every year. We now have a rule that every time anyone starts singing, you have to stand up. It becomes a game everyone can get into and keeps your focus on the thing you're watching.

Sometimes, we just need to give ourselves permission to have some fun and play along. If you have kids, get out there with them and run around, and not just after them (though that I know can be a workout!). Even if you don't have kids, find the nearest playground and hop on one of the swings. You forget how many different part of your body you have to use just to stay seated and get a little air. And again, if you like dancing, as I do, you can throw yourself a mini dance party. Put on three to four of your favorite songs and dance like no one's watching. It's a great way to get in a 10-minute cardio workout, and who doesn't get energized by listening to their favorite jam?

YOUR FITSTYLE PLAN:

This chart will help you move from good ideas to a good plan. The first column is for things you like to do. Anything. If it's knitting, or if it's watching TV, write it down. In the next column, write down the exercises you like to do. Are they walking, swimming, yoga…? You want to be aware of activities that you already enjoy doing. Then, you can consider ways to bring fitness into those activities. You want to start with these things. There's no need to force yourself to do something you don't really like doing.

The last column is for exercise tools that you already own. These are hand weights, a mat, resistance bands, etc.

NON-EXERCISE ACTIVITIES YOU LIKE TO DO:	EXERCISES YOU LIKE TO DO:	EXERCISE TOOLS YOU HAVE AT HOME:

Think about what you like doing. Who do you like hanging out with? How can you combine these with fitness activities?

Use this chart as a reference guide for how you can enjoy yourself while still exercising!

This chart can help you create what I call the 10-10 Rule and be a useful motivator. You pick one of your favorite activities and pair it with an exercise, then you do the activity for 10-minutes followed by the exercise for 10-minutes. One of my friends loves to read and uses this rule when she's on her stationary bike, so she reads for 10-minutes and then cycles like crazy for 10-minutes. It's important that with this rule that you can put 100% of your attention in to the exercise.

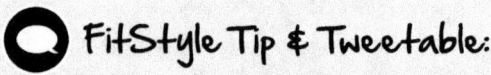 FitStyle Tip & Tweetable:

If it's fun, then I'll run. **#FITSTYLE**

KEY #4

STAGE YOUR LIVING SPACES

OUT OF SIGHT, OUT OF MIND.

Do you own a set of hand weights? If your answer is yes, take a second to conjure up the image of where they are. They usually get relegated to a closet or the basement, where you may keep some other exercise tools that are collecting dust. For a long time, I kept my hand weights under the couch, and at some point when I was cleaning or friends came over, I pushed them in a little further. They rolled just far enough out of my reach that I forgot about them completely.

Does any of this sound familiar to you? Just like how we changed our perspective on exercising (it doesn't have to be a pain!), this key will open a new way to look at our living spaces. We think that because they are exercise tools, we should keep them in the gym or in the area where we "work out", but the problem with that is we may not be in that space very often. The harder we make something for ourselves, the less likely it is we're going to do it. I find we suffer from what I call Out of Sight, Out of Mind Syndrome. You may have every intention of using those hand weights, but because they're somewhere tucked away or simply out of sight, you forget about them.

We need to bring our exercise tools out of those dark confines and put them not only within eyesight, but within reach. You're going to be much more inclined to do a set of bicep curls when you have weights or resistance bands right in front of you.

For example, if you're watching TV or you're in your living room, put your exercise tools, like hand weights or a yoga block, in a basket near your TV. You're much more likely to pick them up because they're right there. You're going to see them, and you're going to walk by them.

Think about your clothing. If you know you're going to head to the gym the next day, put your gym clothes out the night before, or if you want to take a walk when you get back from the office, put your walking shoes right by the door. You want to stage your living spaces so all the props you need are placed as cues and reminders for you to stay active.

Using this mindset, take a walk around your house or office, looking for places and furniture that can act as cues or be used for fitness. I walked around my office looking for places that I could use as a stand up desk. I found a great mantle above an old, non-working fireplace that was a perfect height for me! At the time, I worked in an old renovated mansion. I know. A fireplace is kind of surprising to have in an office. Are there tables or bookshelves where you can use your laptop or even prop up a tablet like an iPad so you can have the screen as close to eye level as possible?

If you have a balance ball, why not roll it into your living room for seating or swap out that office chair?

Many of us spend so much time at the office that we consider it one of our living spaces. If you don't have one already, look into getting a standing desk. There are companies that make accessories to easily retrofit a desk, allowing you to choose between standing or being seated. When you walk into a room, look around and see if there are any high-top tables where you can stand. If you spend a lot of time on the phone, get yourself a wireless headset so you can move around while on a call.

Remember, you're the director and stage manager for your set — and that includes your house, car, office, and anywhere else you spend time.

YOUR FITSTYLE PLAN

Get out the list of exercise tools you completed in the previous section. Go over each one and note how you will move it into eyesight and within reach. Then do it starting with making at least one change right now!

Pack a bag of fitness clothes, complete with shoes, and leave it in your car or in the office. This way you'll always be ready if the opportunity should arise for you to get to a fitness class or take a walk.

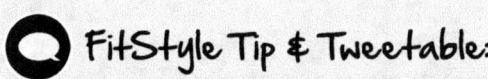 FitStyle Tip & Tweetable:

Whatever your home décor style, fitness is a perfect accessory. **#FITSTYLE**

BONUS TIP:
Smart decorating takes fitness into account. **#FITSTYLE**

KEY #5

BE THANKFUL

IT'S ALL ABOUT THE DETAILS.

Have you ever woken up on the wrong side of the bed? You get out feeling sluggish and maybe a bit depressed, and wish you could lie back down and get out on the other side feeling energized and happy? While that exact method may not work, this next and final key to FitStyle Your Life may be the closest thing to helping you do just that.

The key is to be thankful. I know, you're probably wondering what exactly does this have to do with exercise and fitness. Here's the thing — actively being thankful or showing gratitude addresses our mental fitness, which in turn helps provide the motivation we need to move our bodies and do all the things required of us throughout the day.

Science-backed studies show that people who are thankful:

- **Fall asleep faster and sleep more deeply.** Sleep is essential to allow our bodies to recharge each day.

- **Are happier people.** When those rain clouds come, and they always do, we know to get out the umbrella and keep walking until the sun comes out again.

When we think about fitness as making ourselves strong, it needs to be not just in the physical sense, but also in our mindset. When we work on being thankful, it's like building a muscle, so when something heavy comes our way, we have the strength to make it through or lift it off of us.

When you're happier, you're healthier. It's true. You also have more motivation to move. According to a 2012 study published in *Personality and Individual Differences,* grateful people experience fewer aches and pains, and they also report feeling healthier than other people. Not surprisingly, grateful people are also more likely to take care of their health.

What's important to remember is this is something to get into the habit of doing every day. It's not going to do you much good to confine it to a day or one month in November each year. You know what I'm talking about.

Here's the secret to really making this work: be specific about what you're thankful for.

An example — you might say something like, "I'm thankful for my job." Okay, great, but go the extra step and ask why. What specific thing related to your job are you thankful about, or what happened that you're thankful for?

Here's what I would say: I'm thankful for my boss who gave me an article recently on standing desks because he knows about my interest in bringing fitness into our everyday lives.

Maybe you'd say: "I'm thankful for my cat." I'd push you to say something more like: "I'm thankful for that cute way she purrs when I pet her behind her ears."

So, now it's your turn.

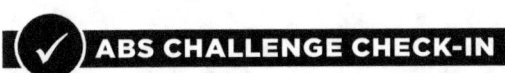

ABS CHALLENGE CHECK-IN

But first, how about a quick check-in? Are your abs still getting a workout? I know you're thankful for this reminder, right?

YOUR FITSTYLE PLAN

Stand up, if you're not already, and take 10 minutes to write down 5 things you're thankful for. They don't have to be connected, but it may make it easier to get into the details that way.

1. _____

2. _____

3. _____

4. _____

5. _____

I'm a big supporter of keeping a gratitude journal for several reasons. It gets you into the habit of thinking about what you're thankful for. It's an awesome recap of your year. I've taken to reading my journal usually around the 6-month mark and then at the end of the year. It's amazing how uplifting it is to be reminded of these little blessings or happy occurrences. Writing regularly, even if it's just one thing daily, helps us to further develop our discipline and follow through, which is helpful for so many other parts of our lives, too.

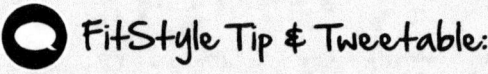 **FitStyle Tip & Tweetable:**

A secret to getting better sleep: get rid of the sheep and count your blessings. **#FITSTYLE**

WHAT'S NEXT?

I hope you've found these 5 keys to FitStyle Your Life helpful:

1. Stand up for your own good.

2. Make every second count.

3. Enjoy yourself.

4. Stage your living spaces.

5. Be thankful.

Before you put this book down, commit to using at least one of these keys and start right now. Which one will you use to start unlocking your personal FitStyle?

I'd love to hear which one you chose and for all of us to keep encouraging one another.

Connect with Me and Others in the ZoeFit Community

FACEBOOK: www.facebook.com/zoefit

TWITTER: www.twitter.com/_zoefit

INSTAGRAM: www.instagram.com/zoefit_style

Tell me which FitStyle key you plan to use by posting a comment on one of these channels or email me directly at **shana@zoefit.com**.

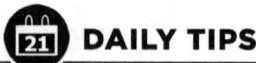 **DAILY TIPS**

If you want reminders on how to implement these keys in your everyday life, sign up for my daily tips. I'll text you with a short tip each day. Just text "zoedaily" to 99-000.

Your data rates will apply, but you can cancel at anytime. To learn more about the daily tips, visit *http://zoefit.com/fitstyle-your-life/daily-tips/*

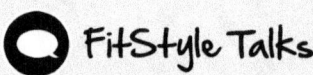 FitStyle Talks

Shana is available for corporate wellness programs and public speaking engagements. She presents interactive and informative talks to large and small groups, incorporating both facts and fitness with audience participation. Learn more at **www.zoefit.com/fitstyle-your-life/talks**

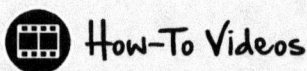 How-To Videos

Watch videos for easy tips, workouts, and decor ideas. Learn more about how to FitStyle Your Life at **www.zoefit.com.**

ABOUT THE AUTHOR

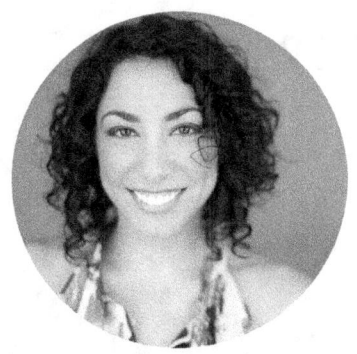

Photo by Steve DePino Photography

Shana N. Schneider is the Founder of ZoeFit and the "FitStyle Your Life" approach. With nearly a decade in the fitness industry, she is passionate about sharing the tips and insights she has learned along the way to help anyone who struggles to find the time for exercise. As a fitness expert, Shana has been featured in national magazines, websites and fitness blogs including The Huffington Post, Redbook, Hella Wella, and MomTrends.com. She has been seen on WTNH News 8 and WTIC FOX-TV CT and Our Lives News 12 Connecticut.

Shana is also a Senior Program Manager for Technolutions. She is an AFAA certified group fitness instructor and holds a B.A. from Yale University.

She's known for doing leg lifts in line at Starbucks and working on her abs while getting a mani pedi.

REFERENCES

PHOTO CREDITS:

Spine Image: https://commons.wikimedia.org/wiki/File:Illu_vertebral_column.jpg

Banana Image: Spotless banana in process of decompose photo by exopixel from DepositPhotos

REFERENCE LINKS:

http://www.mayoclinic.org/healthy-lifestyle/adult-health/expert-answers/sitting/faq-20058005

http://www.health.harvard.edu/blog/much-sitting-linked-heart-disease-diabetes-premature-death-201501227618

http://www.juststand.org/tabid/816/default.aspx

http://www.ncbi.nlm.nih.gov/pmc/articles/PMC4454645/

http://www.ncbi.nlm.nih.gov/pmc/articles/PMC3827429/

http://lifehacker.com/5925428/how-many-hours-you-should-limit-your-sitting-to-to-avoid-an-early-death

http://greatist.com/health/ultimate-guide-good-posture

http://www.ncbi.nlm.nih.gov/pubmed/20543754

http://www.health.ny.gov/diseases/chronic/cvd.htm

http://www.livescience.com/14835-attention-exercise-haters-everyday-activities-improve-fitness.html

http://www.livescience.com/26772-short-exercise-bouts-benefit-health.html

http://well.blogs.nytimes.com/2014/12/10/one-minute-workout/?_r=0

https://www.templeton.org/grateful

http://greatergood.berkeley.edu/expandinggratitude